SOBRIETY:

WINNING OVER ADDICTION

BY

FOY O. PRAIZ

Table Of Content

Introduction

Substance abuse disorder is a worldwide epidemic. It can be devastating to individuals, their loved ones, and their professional endeavours. Illusion plays a crucial role in addiction, leading addicts to believe they are experiencing pleasure when they are not. Addiction is a stigmatizing behavior, and no one enjoys the rejection and scorns they receive because of it.

Despite appearances, addiction is treatable and recoverable with the right help. Continuing to abstain from substances is an essential part of the healing process. To be sober is to abstain from using drugs or alcohol. It's the bedrock of a happy, sober existence.

Addiction cessation is only the first step in sobriety. This trip calls for a radical change in how you live and think. Our goal in writing "Sobriety: A winning over Addiction" is to serve as a thorough resource for anyone just starting on the road to recovery. In this manual, we discuss the value of abstinence, the difficulties associated with it, and methods for overcoming them. We hope to give people a realistic and workable plan for overcoming addiction and finding happiness in recovery. Therefore, this book is for you if you are thinking about sobriety or if you have already started down this road. Come along with us as we learn about sobriety and help you get sober for a better future.

Chapter One

Misperceptions About Sobriety

The goal of therapy for drug and alcohol addiction is commonly described as sobriety, but does it stop there? Sobriety is frequently thought of as when someone completely abstains from particular actions or substances, but in reality, the term refers to abstinence.

According to the majority of academic definitions, sobriety is simply the absence of intoxication at any given time.

There are frequently many assumptions about sobriety that are the consequence of preconceived conceptions, some of which include:

- Being sober is a rather boring activity.

This might be the largest of them all. People frequently worry that if they stop taking drugs or alcohol, they won't ever be able to fully enjoy life again. They frequently fear losing their enthusiasm, flow, or confidence. They worry they won't be able to participate in the former activities that gave them joy. They are worried about losing out on the fun of using or drinking.

While it's true that some drugs might make you feel happier than you would normally, fun and pleasure are different.

Drugs can be so pricey that they can kill someone if they are used only for pleasure. The amount of fun you have in life depends on your thoughts and deeds. Once you've conquered your addiction, you'll have more control over those things. Addiction keeps you performing the same routine with the same negative feeling no matter what you do; it is never exciting or satisfying. Sobriety gives you the freedom to accomplish more things that are intriguing.

- The friends will go.

In reality, you don't need friends who push you toward addictions around, to begin with, and this dread seems to be the root of most people's anxiety. Most often, they are shocked to discover that their only things in common with those friends were drug and alcohol abuse. Even while it can be difficult to acknowledge, it's evidence that they weren't friends in the first place because those that genuinely care about you will want the best for you.

- In the mirror, you won't recognize yourself.

Some people's viewpoints have evolved as a result of alcohol and drug use over time to the point that they now think that's who they are. For some, it serves as a coping mechanism for social acceptance, thus giving it up makes them feel as though they are losing their identity. Using drugs and alcohol does not represent a true identity; rather, it is frequently evidence of a false identity.

Co-dependent relationships, in which individuals repress their own identities to please those around them, are also created as a result of addictions. This is because addiction is a disease of the brain. One of the first steps in recovering from substance misuse is discovering your true identity.

It's conceivable that you have other preconceived views about sobriety that keep you from fully dedicating yourself to the healing process. It is crucial to be aware of these presumptions and to carefully assess if any actual evidence exists to support them. The sooner you discover this and get rid of them, the better your recuperation will be because they don't usually.

- Simply put, those who are addicted are unable to regulate their conduct.

It is commonly believed that those who are dependent on drugs or alcohol lack the resolve to stop using them, but addiction alters the brains of users in ways that make it very difficult for them to exercise self-control and willpower. It becomes challenging to abstain from consuming the substance as a result. Drug abuse results in the production of chemicals in the brain linked to pleasure, which over time alters the regions of the brain that are in charge of motivation, pleasure, and memory. As a result, cravings are triggered, leading users to prioritize drug use over other activities.

What is Self-Awareness?

The state of being aware of one's thoughts, behaviours, and feelings in various circumstances is known as self-awareness. Being fully aware of oneself, including how one reacts to various situations, persons, and settings, is the condition of self-awareness. Self-awareness is the antithesis of denial, which many addicts experience when unaware of their addiction's seriousness.

It can be difficult to maintain a healthy level of self-awareness as a result of ongoing substance usage, especially when attempting to stop using substances. This underlines once more how crucial self-awareness is when undergoing therapy.

Self-awareness's function in sobriety

Self-awareness and sobriety have the potential to produce amazing results when combined. For a variety of reasons, including some of the following, it is crucial to retain a high level of self-awareness to successfully recover from addiction:

- It encourages altruism.

The practice of active self-awareness will reveal addiction as a type of selfishness. Whether or not someone wants to be that way, addiction has a way of bringing out the worst in them. This mental disease promotes pursuing personal gain while ignoring the welfare of others.

- It encourages independence and uniqueness.

Looking for outside support and aid seems sensible when going through a trying circumstance. However, while you work through the recovery process from addiction, you could find that you rely on a few people more than usual to get you through the day. This type of conduct is undesirable for both parties, but it also fosters dependency, which is a surefire path to relapse. On the other side, self-awareness encourages independence and constantly reminds you that you are the only one who can maintain your sobriety.

- It helps you make the distinction between good and bad.

Knowing yourself better enables you to discern between the triggers for your addiction and those that do not.

- Aware of oneself while moving

Considerable thought must be given to the following to achieve self-awareness:

i. Determine the cause or origin of the addiction.
ii. Live in the present and forget the past.
iii. Keep a daily journal recording your progress.
iv. Have a buddy to hold you accountable.
v. Be impartial; avoid being irrational.
vi. Recognize your emotions, and don't be afraid to express them.
vii. Recognize any patterns of conduct that may have contributed to the emergence of your addiction, no matter how unimportant.

Chapter Two

Setting and achieving sobriety-related goals

The road to sobriety is made simpler and quicker by understanding one's relationship with all types of addiction. Additionally, it establishes the foundations for ongoing self-care, social support, and new habits that could help with mental refocus.

Addiction begins with a relatively small act (such as social interaction, sleep disorders treatment, stress management techniques, etc.) and develops sporadically until it spirals out of control. In most circumstances, it has several significant downsides and does little to allay these worries in the long run.

You may find the following ideas helpful in creating a viable plan:

i.   Look into how it affects people's health.

There are several ways that substance misuse can harm a person's health. For instance, consuming alcohol in moderation may have mild side effects like drowsiness, fogginess, and hangovers; continuing to do so will have detrimental effects on one's health, including disturbed sleep, digestive issues, memory issues, increased anxiety, sadness, and irritability, arguments, and other forms of conflict with loved ones. If these problems are not addressed, they may develop into more serious problems.

Even if recovering from addiction is not a full-time profession, one can get a handle on the issue by continuously analysing their behaviours.

ii.   Prudence management

This plan's major objective is to gradually lower each person's consumption of alcoholic beverages, illegal substances, and other connected things. Investigating one's connection with alcohol is how it is done.

To accomplish this,

a.   Decide why you are doing it. The first and most crucial step in giving up anything is to do this.

b.   Determine how much fluids you consume each day. Consider your motivations for drinking and your triggers, which may include things like relationship stress, social situations, issues at work, or insomnia.

  c. Analyse-it thoroughly: By being open and honest about your feelings towards alcohol, you may encourage others to reflect on their drinking behaviours. It will also boost individual motivation and accountability.

iii. Create or join a community.

Making connections with people who hold the same beliefs about leading a life free from addiction can be very helpful. Remove any evidence of triggers from your home completely. alluring.

Chapter Three

Applications of emotional intelligence

What exactly is EQ or emotional intelligence?

The capacity to recognize, use, and regulate your own emotions to reduce stress, communicate, sympathize with others, overcome obstacles, and diffuse conflict is known as emotional intelligence (EQ). You can develop stronger relationships, perform well at work and school, and reach your professional and personal objectives with the aid of emotional intelligence. Additionally, it can assist you in establishing a connection with your emotions, putting your intentions into practice, and choosing what is most important to you.

Four characteristics are frequently used to characterize emotional intelligence:

Self-management: You can restrain impulsive thoughts, feelings, and actions; healthily regulate your emotions; take the initiative; top your world.

Self-awareness: You are aware of your feelings and how they influence your decisions and actions. You are confident in yourself and are aware of your talents and flaws.

Social awareness: You are socially aware and compassionate. You can discern emotional indicators, comprehend the needs and worries of others, feel at ease in social situations, and comprehend the power relationships in a team or organization.

Relationship management: skills include the ability to establish and maintain positive connections, speak effectively, motivate and influence others, function well in a team, and control conflict.

What makes emotional IQ so crucial?

The most prosperous or contented individuals are not necessarily the most intelligent. There are several instances of people who excel intellectually yet struggle socially and are unproductive at work or in their relationships. To succeed in life, one needs more than just a strong mind. Success in the truest sense is defined by the fluid relationships between these quotients.

i. Physical Performance: Emotional intelligence reduces social difficulties in the workplace and equips one to be a leader and an inspiration to others. Employees now place emotional intelligence over technical skills.

ii. Physical health: Lack of emotional intelligence will result in major health issues like high blood pressure, a weakened immune system, heart attacks and strokes, infertility, and ageing in a time when there are so many external stimuli that can stress the body. Learning how to control your stress is the first step to increasing your emotional intelligence.

iii. Mental health: The inability to control one's emotions makes one more susceptible to anxiety and sadness. Lack of ability to comprehend, feel at ease with, or control one's emotions will lead to loneliness and isolation, which is the main contributor to mental health issues.

iv. Relationships: Developing emotional intelligence affects the ability to express one's thoughts and feelings freely. As a result, relationships all around the world become stronger and communication becomes more effective.

v. social intelligence: Understanding your emotions helps you connect with others and the environment around you on a social level.

How to increase emotional intelligence

• Self-control

You must be able to use your emotions to guide wise decisions about your behaviour if you want to employ your EQ. Overstress might make it difficult for you to maintain control over your emotions and make wise decisions.

Emotions are significant indicators of who you are and what you are like, but when faced with stress that pushes us beyond our comfort zones, we may get overwhelmed and lose control of our emotions. You can learn to take in painful information without allowing it to take control of your thoughts and self-control if you can moderate your tension and remain emotionally present. You'll be able to make decisions that help you maintain emotional control, take initiative, keep your word when you commit to something, and adjust to changing circumstances.

• Self-awareness

Building emotional intelligence requires more than just being able to manage stress. According to the science of attachment, your current emotional state is probably a reflection of what you went through in infancy. Your capacity for controlling fundamental emotions like sadness, joy, fear, and rage is frequently influenced by the calibre and constancy of your early emotional experiences. Your emotions are probably valuable assets in adult life if your primary caregiver as an infant recognized and cherished them. However, if you had perplexing, frightening, or painful emotional experiences as a baby, you may have made an effort to suppress your feelings.

But the secret to knowing how emotion affects your ideas and actions is being able to connect to your emotions—having a moment-to-moment connection with your shifting emotional experience. You must acknowledge, embrace, and get comfortable with your fundamental emotions if you want to develop emotional intelligence (EQ) and become emotionally healthy. This is something that mindfulness practice can help you with.

Focusing on the present moment on purpose and without passing judgment is the practice of mindfulness. Buddhism is where the practice of mindfulness originated, but similar forms of prayer or meditation are practised by the majority of world religions. With the use of mindfulness, you may change your focus from being preoccupied with thoughts to appreciating the present, and your physical and emotional experiences, and gaining a wider perspective on life. As you become more focused and at peace, you become more self-aware.

• Social conscience

You can identify and decipher the primarily nonverbal clues that people use to communicate with you by having social awareness. These indicators enable you to understand how others are genuinely feeling, how their emotional state shifts over time, and what matters most to them.

You can read and comprehend the power dynamics and shared emotional experiences of a group when they exhibit similar nonverbal clues. Simply said, you're socially confident and sympathetic.

You must comprehend the significance of mindfulness in the social process if you want to develop social awareness. After all, when you're lost in your thoughts, distracted by other thoughts, or just zoning out on your phone, you can't pick up on tiny nonverbal signs. Your present-day awareness is necessary for social awareness. While many of us take pleasure in our ability to multitask, doing so means you'll miss the subtle emotional changes that other people are going through and how those changes might help you completely comprehend them.

Putting other thoughts aside and concentrating on the contact itself increases your chances of achieving your social objectives.

To follow the flow of another person's emotional reactions, you must also be aware of the changes in your own emotional experience.

The ability to focus on others does not mean that you are less aware of yourself. You may learn a lot about yourself, your values, and your views by taking the time and making the effort to listen to people. For instance, you would have discovered something significant about yourself if you find it uncomfortable when hearing others voice particular viewpoints.

• Relationship administration

Beginning the process of working productively with others requires emotional awareness and the capacity to identify and comprehend what other people are going through. Once emotional awareness is present, you can effectively learn new social and emotional skills that will improve the quality, quantity, and effectiveness of your interactions.

Learn to be conscious of your nonverbal communication skills. The numerous muscles in your face, particularly those in the area surrounding your eyes, nose, lips, and forehead, allow you to read the emotions of others and express your feelings without using words. Even if you choose to disregard the signals from your emotional brain, others won't. Relationship improvement can be greatly aided by being aware of the nonverbal cues you convey to others.

Play and have fun to de-stress. Play, laughing, and humour are all effective stress relievers. They lighten your load and assist you in maintaining perspective. Laughter balances your neurological system, lowering tension, calming you down, focusing your thinking, and increasing your capacity for empathy.

Recognize that disagreements can bring people closer together. In human interactions, conflict and disagreement are unavoidable. It is impossible for two people to always have the same wants, beliefs, and expectations. That needn't be a terrible thing, though. Building trust among people can result from conflict resolution that is productive and healthy. Conflict encourages freedom, creativity, and safety in relationships when it is not seen as threatening or punishing.

Chapter Four

Understanding Triggers and Cravings

Depending on how you handle them, triggers and cravings will either make recovery easier or harder. A trigger is anything that causes the brain to associate an unpleasant thought, emotion, or memory with addiction.

The desire for food and the desire for drugs or alcohol are extremely similar. Cravings are a typical aspect of addiction and do not indicate relapse when they occur. Individuals have different ways of describing cravings; they may describe them as a pit-like feeling in the stomach, a racing heart, an illusory flavour, etc. Throughout the procedure, cravings will fluctuate in intensity and level.

recognizing the difference between triggers and cravings

The main contrast between appetites and triggers is the level of dimension somebody possesses. Triggers frequently involve ideas or recollections. Cravings have a heightened emotional, mental, and physical impact. Additionally, a need may manifest even when you are not exposed to the trigger.

Because a craving is a passing want, it can be satisfied. Recognizing, understanding, and waiting for the craving to pass will help you manage it. As a self-control mechanism is created, cravings become less intense, which has a significant impact on recovery. When one puts in the effort, allows patience, receives some instruction, and receives encouragement, cravings are easily overcome.

Managing circumstances that cause triggers

Understanding the causes of the emotional reactions felt is necessary to manage triggers during addiction recovery;

doing so will motivate one to work toward emotional liberation.

Additionally, identifying the emotional response as soon as it appears physically in the body will aid in rehabilitation. Once you are aware of a trigger and the response it causes in you, the next step is to change your emotional state.

Any addiction that is being treated must be able to be overcome. Patients must receive instruction from the program on how to keep their sobriety over the long term. At the beginning of their recovery journey, a person may be able to become sober on their own, but it is extremely improbable that they will be able to maintain their sobriety without any help. To effectively manage intrusive thoughts, overcome withdrawal symptoms, and maintain an inner calm, one must develop healthy coping skills while in therapy.

One of the most difficult components of overcoming addiction and sustaining a long-lasting recovery is learning to control triggers and cravings. It is also among the most crucial elements.

Triggers are stimuli that serve as reminders of a person's prior substance usage.

The term "triggered" in daily life describes the emergence of an unpleasant emotional experience in reaction to a specific stimulus as a result of a prior painful experience with that particular catalyst. In a similar vein, triggers are the stimuli that are most likely to result in emotional distress.

Triggers are things that act as reminders of situations where substance use was prevalent during the process of recovering from addiction. An anxiety attack may be sparked by someone, something, a place, a smell, a situation, or simply a distant notion. When seeking to understand what triggers are, it can be beneficial to think of them as either internal or external impulses.

One example of an external addiction trigger is a stressful or unhappy history.

ii. Being in the company of habitual drug users.

iii. Having access to people you can ask to buy alcohol or other substances for you.

iv. Social gatherings where using drugs and alcohol is accepted or encouraged.

v. Smells that conjure up memories of your prior drug use.

vi. Financial difficulties

vii. Trauma

Internal triggers, unlike external triggers, are typically emotional low points that raise the chance of relapse. A plentiful supply of internal boost is having happy memories of one's past substance.

Some specific instances of elements that may serve as internal addiction triggers include the following:

i. Depression
ii. A distressed mental state.
iii. Feelings of being overwhelmed.
iv. Thinking back on joyful life experiences "just like everyone else."
v. Anniversary of substance abuse
vi. The resurfacing of unresolved unpleasant memories

In addition to functioning as reminders of past drug-related events, triggers can significantly contribute to the beginning of cravings.

Cravings are a motivating factor in both using and abstaining from substances when they occur in the context of recovery. Cravings can be either a mental or physical desire to use substances. It can occur at any moment, anywhere, or even in response to the slightest notion of using drugs. It is incredibly unexpected. Cravings are another typical withdrawal symptom that people go through when they try to reduce or stop using their preferred substance.

Most of the time, no one is born with a need for material; instead, it begins when both the mind and body begin to yearn for something more than what is considered "normal functioning". When alcohol or drugs are consumed, dopamine, a hormone secreted during pleasure, is released excessively into the brain (this results in a feeling of euphoria that, over time, causes the brain to crave its excessive amount), leading the respondent to continue using drugs as a way to satiate that craving.

Recovery is a long process that requires a lot of patience to finish and maintain. The pleasurable and motivational alterations brought on by recurrent substance use require some time for the brain to undo.

The following are some instances of typical drug and alcohol cravings:

i.   Irresistible physical urges to use.
ii. Constantly thinking about a substance.

iii. The desire to feel the positive mental or physical consequences that drug use can produce.

iv. A desire for something out of the ordinary.

v. You feel intense emotional distress when you think about the drug.

Learning how to control the factors that lead to cravings is essential during addiction therapy. Everybody will experience a different variety of triggers and urges, so understanding the triggers can help you better manage the appetites they produce.

Addiction treatment centres offer a range of cognitive, behavioural, holistic, and experiential therapies. Patients who undergo these treatments learn a variety of complementary strategies for avoiding and conquering cravings and triggers.

Addiction treatment also teaches techniques to create healthy coping skills to employ in circumstances of negative emotions, which lowers the likelihood of relapsing in the future.

Cravings can fluctuate in both duration and intensity. Some desires may only last a brief period, while others may last many days or even longer. After the high wears off, a person can get a hunger right away, or it might take them another 30 years to notice.

Chapter Five

The Escape

Any type of addiction recovery needs both personal development and several deliberate developmental techniques to reduce the likelihood of relapsing at any stage while in recovery.

The following are typical causes of relapse:

a) Boredom
b) Stress
c) Financial Problems
d) Interpersonal Relationship Issues
e) Special Sights and Smells
f) Special People or Places
g) Going back to old habits
h) Anger

Rehab or addiction treatment facilities educate patients on relapse prevention techniques to support clients in maintaining their recovery and achieving both short- and long-term objectives.

To lower the risk of relapsing, a variety of relapse prevention techniques can be included in daily activities. Every individual in recovery should incorporate these techniques into their daily schedule and routine to minimize or at the very least low the chances of cravings.

They consist of:

• **Self-care**

Two of the most typical post-acute withdrawal symptoms that addicts have are insomnia and tiredness. Regular physical activity, leading a healthy lifestyle, and eating a balanced diet can all help to enhance sleep quality. Establishing and maintaining a schedule for one's eating, sleeping, and exercise behaviours can help with this. By doing this, one can retrain their body to sleep better, which will also assist lower the likelihood that they would relapse into their previous patterns.

• **HALT** (Hungry, Angry, Lonely, and Tired) is an abbreviation that stands for asking questions when feeling these emotions. It will help to ask specific questions if there is a desire to use anything when one is feeling anxious or "off" in general. For those undergoing addiction treatment, the most frequent triggers are hunger, rage, loneliness, and fatigue. Taking the HALT inventory can help reduce the likelihood of relapsing into old behaviours if it is observed.

• **Meditation**

Another type of mental exercise that promotes self-awareness is the practice of mindfulness meditation. A sense of self-awareness offers one an advantage against elements that can cause relapse. The combination of aspects like acceptance, giving up control, as well as prayer and meditation, characterizes the practice of mindfulness meditation.

The core of the mindfulness notion is the meditation practice regarding oneself and the surroundings. The first step toward cultivating greater mindfulness is awareness without judgment. It might be beneficial to increase one's awareness of what they are doing, thinking, and feeling in the present moment by writing down their everyday activities or keeping track of them using a smartphone. When overcoming cravings, this might result in important insights and a sense of empowerment.

• Awareness of Personal Triggers

Triggers are people, places, or things that conjure up past uses. Triggers can be internal or external, such as anxiety, impatience, stress, wrath, and low self-esteem. Writing down both internal and external triggers and keeping the list handy is one of the best strategies to become aware of one's triggers and lower the risk of relapsing.

• Joining a peer-helping initiative.

It is really helpful to participate regularly in a support group that assists you, holds you accountable, educates you, and gives you the chance to connect with others who can relate to what you are going through. The use of peer support and having a sponsor can be highly beneficial to a recovery program. It lessens the likelihood of isolation and loneliness, both of which can serve as relapse triggers. This is yet another method that aids in relapse prevention by avoiding relapse.

• Grounding Methods

The biggest obstacles to a full recovery are typically stress and anxiety. The grounding approach, often known as the "5-4-3-2-1 coping technique," can be a useful tool for lowering the likelihood of subsequent relapse. It entails focusing on the 'now and now' with the help of the five senses rather than using narcotics or other methods that could lead to relapse.

Take a few deep, steady breaths as you begin the first of the five steps.

5: Visualize five objects in your immediate surroundings.

4. List four nearby items that you can reach with your hand.

3. Identify three distinct sounds that are happening nearby.

2: Name the two distinct odours that you can detect in the region.

1 Identify one flavour you can taste in your surroundings.

Take a couple more slow, deep breaths to complete this exercise. By concentrating on your senses, which will help you feel more in control and less overwhelmed, you may complete everyday chores, overcome unhealthy thoughts or feelings, feel more in control and less overwhelmed, and lower the risk of relapse.

Deep breathing exercises can also help you become more mindful and aware of yourself.

The most crucial aspect of existence is breathing; altering one's breathing patterns will have a big impact on their quality of life. Breathing affects a wide range of essential bodily processes that take place throughout the body and the chemical composition of the brain.

Deep breathing triggers the release of neurotransmitters in the brain that then trigger the production of feel-good hormones, causing sensations of relaxation, happiness, and a decrease in pain. Deep breathing increases the flow of oxygen throughout the body as well as encourages the body to release toxins. For deep breathing, the 4 by 4 breathing practice is useful. Inhale deeply for four breaths via your nose, hold each for four seconds, and then slowly exhale. You should be able to feel your diaphragm contracting and expanding as you breathe. Deep breathing is a great relapse prevention strategy since you can perform it in almost any place and no one will ever know that you are doing it.

• **Sincerity and Accountability**.

Being held accountable to someone else will go a great way in helping to conquer the temptation for former substances in the early stages of recovery when fighting it might be difficult. These people will be resolute in their desire to enforce tight discipline over abandoning the conduct while remaining non-judgmental.

A skill that can be very helpful in preventing relapses is compiling a list of clean and healthy family members and friends who are also going through treatment and whom you can call for assistance.

Get Support

Although the worry of reverting to previous behaviours can be paralyzing, this shouldn't necessarily be the case given the abundance of coping mechanisms available. It will be possible to entirely eradicate the dread by reaching out to those who have experienced similar circumstances and by obtaining medical advice.

Chapter Six

Nutrition and Exercise for Complete Recovery
Physical Activity

Consistent physical activity will achieve similar goals, aiding the body in its recuperation, whether it be high-intensity workouts like jogging for miles or low-impact exercises like walking around the block. It triggers the body's natural defence against the onset of depression, the hormone "Endorphin," to be released.

Beyond its physical advantages, exercise allows for social connection, which will hasten the recovery from any type of addiction. Individuals should select a hobby they will like doing for the rest of their lives because continuity is the foundation of any real change. Exercise shouldn't be done too regularly though, as this might lead to the dry drunk syndrome, which is characterized by the persistence of addictive behavioural patterns despite the absence of substance usage.

Notably, addiction can spread to other activities like hobbies or task-oriented activities like exercise in addition to the use of illegal substances.

Nutrition

Recovery depends in large measure on proper nutrition. Major nutrients of sufficient quality are required to fill the void that was caused by the usage of drugs. A balanced diet that includes items like oranges, avocados, berries, green vegetables, legumes, and certain grains is advised.

Diets high in nutrients like amino acids (which release dopamine) and low in glycaemic carbohydrates are advised for a rapid recovery. Sugary foods and caffeinated beverages should be avoided to prevent relapse.

Exercise and nutrition are important because:

i. Healthy feelings will automatically be promoted by food selection and exercise. When diet and exercise are given top priority, benefits such as weight loss, improved health and well-being, and a decreased risk of major health issues due to substance misuse are attained.

ii. It is simpler to achieve goals and add order to daily life when one develops and maintains a balanced diet.

iii. Establishes a sound framework for daily planning, rewiring the brain to focus on elements critical to sobriety's success.

iv. Eases anxiety and decreases stress.

v. Controls sleeping patterns and promotes deep sleep.

Conclusion

The road to recovery from addiction may be long, arduous, and travelled alone, but it is a road that is well worth it. After going through addiction treatment, it can be difficult to remain sober, but there are many different ways that this goal can be accomplished.

 A key part of being able to prevent relapse is being able to recognize the personal factors that can bring it on. Because of this, it is essential to have a solid understanding of the reasons for addiction as well as methods for overcoming its effects.

Achieving sobriety is a process that calls for steadfastness, effort, and dedication on the part of the individual. It needs us to let go of our desire to be flawless and our self-will to say that we are making progress rather than perfecting anything. A daily commitment to sobriety is necessary for successful recovery, which is a process rather than an event.

There are a great many advantages to abstaining from alcohol. It not only liberates us from the shackles of addiction, but it also paves the way for other beneficial transformations in our lives. Achieving recovery is the beginning of a life that is not just free from addiction but also one that is filled with hope, serenity, and joy.